Effects of Alternative and Modern Medicine on Longevity And Healthy Aging

Dr. Patrick Abiuso

TABLE OF CONTENTS

INTRODUCTION

Growing up, I remember hearing the phrase, "When it's your time, it's your time," referring to the timing of one's passing. And I guess that it is a true statement to some degree, but is it also possible that there are factors under our control that affect that timing? And can these factors not only affect how long we live but, even more importantly, influence the quality of our later years? We are going to explore how both alternative medicine and modern medicine play a role in healthy aging and longevity.

I am an internal medicine specialist who has been involved in healthcare for 50 years. I was trained in traditional medicine and have diagnosed and helped many patients with that knowledge. In addition to pharmaceuticals, preventive care, and vaccines, I have also utilized alternative forms of therapy in patient care. I am writing this book to review some of these therapies for people who would like more information on these modalities. Although I am not an herbalist or nutritionist per se, I have been able to incorporate these therapies with some success in my practice, and I will attempt to give the reader an overview of these modalities and how they relate to healthy living as we age and the components of longevity.

We will review some dietary plans and the need for vitamins and minerals in our diet and discuss various herbs. Herbs have many therapeutic uses and are helpful in various medical conditions. Vitamins and minerals play a vital role in human metabolism. Deficiencies cause a number of diseases. Other nontraditional approaches include forms of physical therapy, nutritional counseling, and types of meditation. We will look at practices that promote graceful aging and how we can retard the aging process. And we will look at how modern medicine has affected human mortality.

As always, a patient should discuss alternative therapy plans with their physician after doing their own research. You should take care when choosing supplements, with attention to purity and contamination. Also know that some supplements may interact with medications and may increase or decrease medication potency or enhance side effects. There are not many double-blind studies (where you don't know what you are getting and I, as the researcher, don't know what I am giving you), so some of this information is gained from anecdotal evidence or personal experience. Some is based on observational data. Be wary of advertisers who make claims before doing your own research.

Dietary interventions are associated with reduced risk of many diseases, such as hypertension, diabetes, and cardiovascular disease. Lifestyle modifications, including physical exercise, avoidance of tobacco, limiting alcohol intake, and stress reduction, are important in maintaining cellular and systemic health. Vitamins A, B, C, D, E, and K are important factors in numerous metabolic pathways, including energy production, DNA synthesis, repair, antioxidant defense, and cellular signaling. Minerals that are needed for proper cellular function include sodium, potassium, calcium, magnesium, phosphate, and trace elements such as zinc, copper, cobalt, selenium, and molybdenum. Again, these substances are needed for DNA synthesis as well as many other cellular functions. New areas of research are looking at these substances and their relationship to diabetes by affecting the pancreas and various other metabolic pathways.

CHAPTER 1

Philosophers such as Sigmund Freud, Soren Kierkegaard, and Ernest Becker proposed that awareness of mortality influences much of human behavior and is key to understanding human behavior. I am starting with this thought as a segue into a discussion on aging and how healthy living can affect this process.

Aging is characterized by the progressive loss of physiological integrity. This deterioration is associated with many medical conditions. The rate of aging has not only a genetic component, but also involves molecular changes, cellular communication dysfunction, stem cell depletion, and chronic inflammation, all of which are interrelated and affect the process. Stem cell replacement is being investigated as a way of mitigating these effects, but such treatments are expensive and still investigational. There are challenges concerning sources, delivery, immunogenicity, and long-term side effects. So what are some other safer ways to slow down the aging process?

Free radicals are chemical atoms, molecules, or ions that contain one or more unpaired electrons in their outer orbits, making them highly reactive with other molecules. Some free radicals are useful in cellular metabolism, but others can be produced by environmental toxins, radiation, and inflammation. Excessive production of these substances or insufficient removal can lead to cellular damage by affecting the cell's DNA or the products that DNA produces.

Armed with this knowledge as background, researchers have been looking for substances that can neutralize free radicals in the human body. These substances are known as antioxidants and include vitamins A, C, and E; polyphenols; flavonoids; carotenoids; and other phytochemicals found in fruits, vegetables, and certain plant-derived foods.

Antioxidants work by donating electrons to free radicals, stabilizing them and thereby preventing oxidative damage to cells, DNA, proteins, and lipids, and decreasing oxidative stress. Several studies indicate that diets rich in natural antioxidants are associated with reduced risk of chronic disease.

CHAPTER 2

Using these facts, let's look at some diets that are thought to be associated with beneficial health effects. These diets are rich in plant-based foods and emphasize green leafy vegetables, berries, nuts, olive oil, and whole grains.

The DASH diet (Dietary Approaches to Stop Hypertension) is a dietary plan developed to emphasize foods high in potassium, calcium, and magnesium, while limiting sodium, saturated fats, and cholesterol. The focus is on fruits and vegetables, whole grains, low-fat dairy, and lean protein such as fish and poultry.

The Mediterranean diet is a way of eating based on the traditional diet of people who live in the Mediterranean region of the world. It emphasizes plant-based foods such as vegetables, fruits, whole grains, legumes, and healthy fats like olive oil, and includes limited fish, poultry, dairy, and red meat. There is a social component around meals in this region that is thought to be beneficial.

The MIND diet contains elements of the Mediterranean diet and the DASH diet to promote brain health in an attempt to reduce cognitive decline. It emphasizes foods rich in antioxidants and anti-inflammatory components. Butter, cheese, red meat, fried or fast foods, and sweets are limited.

Why are these diets thought to be healthy for humans? How do they reduce cardiovascular and neurodegenerative diseases? How do they protect cellular integrity and promote longevity? It is because these diets provide a broad spectrum of phytonutrients, antioxidants, and fiber. Natural substances like omega-3 fatty acids are heart-healthy. Polyphenols such as curcumin, quercetin, and flavonoids are found in green leafy vegetables and berries. These substances exert both antioxidant and anti-inflammatory endothelial effects and reduce oxidative stress. Fiber from oats and legumes lowers LDL cholesterol, improving cardiac function. In addition, essential vitamins and botanicals such as ginkgo biloba, bacopa monnieri, and withania somnifera may help cognition. Plant-derived substances such as garlic, green tea, and curcumin have lipid-lowering, antioxidant, and anti-inflammatory properties.

In summary, interventions to retard aging and promote optimal cellular and physiological function include dietary intervention along with vitamins, minerals, and lifestyle modification.

CHAPTER 3

So you might ask, why don't I just eat only healthy fruits and vegetables? It's not that simple, since deficiencies can occur, especially with chronic disease, in the elderly, during pregnancy, etc. Awareness is key in following a healthy diet tailored to yourself. With that as a background, I would like to discuss specific foods and their benefits.

Blueberries contain anthocyanins, which are thought to protect DNA from aging and improve brain function, thereby helping to prevent memory deterioration.

Red meat and fish contain amino acids that form creatine, a compound that promotes ATP production. ATP is a major source of energy for cells. Creatine may enhance athletic performance, and there's some evidence that it may support brain health. Red meat is also a source of iron and vitamin B12, as well as some L-arginine and coenzyme Q10, which are thought to have beneficial effects on heart health.

Avocados contain vitamins C and E, lutein, and glutathione, which prevent damage from free radicals and also have anti-inflammatory effects. These elements improve skin elasticity and help maintain a healthy scalp.

Wild salmon is a source of omega-3 fatty acids and astaxanthin, which fight inflammation and protect the skin from wrinkles.

Dairy foods contain calcium, potassium, vitamins A and D, and protein, all of which are important for bone health and overall body maintenance.

Nuts, like walnuts, may enhance longevity genes and help fight inflammation.

Broccoli is a source of vitamins C and K and lutein, which helps produce collagen and maintain healthy skin.

Lignans, found in foods like lentils, fight free radicals.

Dark leafy greens are a source of folate and vitamin K and aid in bone and muscle metabolism.

Fruits are good sources of vitamins, and pomegranates contain compounds that may help prevent skin wrinkling.

Sweet potatoes are rich in antioxidants and promote digestive and eye health.

Carrots contain fiber, potassium, and vitamins K and A. They help eye health, reduce inflammation, and enhance immunity.

A healthy, balanced diet such as the one described should help maintain good health and proper functioning. Conversely, a diet high in ultra-processed foods, trans fats, sodium, sugary drinks, artificial dyes, and processed meats may accelerate the aging process.

Tomatoes are a source of vitamins A, C, and K and contain lycopene, an antioxidant thought to protect against certain cancers. They also contain lutein and zeaxanthin, which promote healthy eyes.

Plums contain bioactive compounds such as polyphenols and anthocyanins that have shown some anticancer properties. These effects are attributed to antioxidant, anti-inflammatory, and antiangiogenic activity. However, current evidence is primarily from animal studies, and further human studies are needed.

Eggs contain essential nutrients like high-quality protein, choline, vitamin B12, iodine, vitamin D, and selenium, which aid in muscle, bone, and brain health.

Olive oil is a source of healthy monounsaturated fats and lowers the risk of heart disease.

Barley and fiber in general, found in grains, help regulate blood pressure, blood sugar, and digestion.

The allium family, onions, garlic, shallots, leeks, and scallions, contains sulfides and saponins, which help maintain blood pressure and blood sugar levels. They also contain antioxidants with anti-inflammatory properties, making them ideal for patients with autoimmune diseases or arthritis.

Pomegranates are rich in antioxidants, vitamins, minerals, and fiber. They have been used in traditional medicine to treat gastrointestinal issues and are thought to reduce inflammation, fight heart disease, and combat aging.

Watercress contains high levels of antioxidants such as carotenoids, lutein, and zeaxanthin, which protect cells from damage and reduce inflammation. It also contains multiple vitamins and minerals.

Some other helpful dietary hints:

- Drink milk for bone health
- Eat spinach for anemia
- Eat prunes for constipation
- Eat kiwi for insomnia
- Eat parsley for bad breath
- Eat yogurt for good digestion
- Eat turmeric for arthritis
- Eat dark chocolate for anxiety or depression
- A mixture of bananas and rice may help slow diarrhea

Garlic contains compounds including allicin and sulfides, which are believed to have anti-inflammatory, antimicrobial, and heart-protective properties.

Although it is a common belief that cranberry juice cures urinary tract infections because it contains compounds that help prevent bacteria from adhering to the bladder wall, there is no evidence that it is a proven cure.

CHAPTER 4

Now let's turn our attention to vitamins and minerals and review some of their functions and, conversely, what diseases can result from deficiencies. Vitamins are essential compounds that our body needs for growth, development, and overall health. Many vitamins were discovered by studying deficiency diseases in animals. The origin of the word vitamin comes from the Latin word "vita," meaning life. Vitamins transformed medicine by turning mysterious diseases into treatable ones.

We will start with thiamine, or vitamin B1. Sources include meat, milk, citrus fruits, and flour. Beriberi is the disease of thiamine deficiency and can occur with insufficient dietary intake, chronic alcoholism, or ingestion of substances that break it down or interfere with its function, such as large amounts of coffee, tea, or raw shellfish. Thiamine is needed for the nervous system, so symptoms of deficiency can include difficulty walking and numbness of the extremities. It is also helpful for irritability and poor appetite.

Probably the most well-known disease linked to vitamin deficiency is vitamin C deficiency, or scurvy. Sources of vitamin C are fruits and vegetables, and alcoholism is a risk factor. Vitamin C is also important in collagen production and is needed to form healthy skin, endothelial surfaces, and connective tissue structures. In addition, vitamin C aids in iron absorption, so with a deficiency, the patient should also be checked for anemia. Deficiency symptoms may include fatigue, hemorrhages, impaired wound healing (altered immunity), weakness, and problems with the skin and scalp. It is thought that vitamin C may help speed recovery from colds and flu.

Vitamin A is obtained from vegetables, milk, meat, and eggs. Vitamin A is important for vision, and deficiencies can cause visual problems such as night blindness and dry eyes. It can also cause hair loss and affect the skin. This vitamin is also important in enhancing the immune system.

Vegetables, eggs, nuts, and fruits are sources of vitamin E. Vitamin E is important for immunity. Deficiency is uncommon but can affect the neurological and hematological systems. Vitamin E is also helpful in maintaining smooth skin.

Vitamin D helps the body absorb calcium and phosphorus and is essential for building strong bones. A deficiency causes a condition known as rickets, which leads to weakness and deformity of muscles and bones. Fish, eggs, and liver are high in vitamin D. I often advise calcium with vitamin D supplements in patients with osteopenia, especially after menopause.

Vitamin B12 can be obtained from meat, milk, and eggs. It plays an important role in red blood cell production, energy metabolism, and nervous system function. Deficiencies can result in anemia and neuropathy. Folate, found in green leafy vegetables, fruits, and beans, works with B12 in the formation of red blood cells. It is also thought to help with fatigue. I have used these vitamins in patients with certain types of anemia with good results.

Niacin, or vitamin B3, helps convert food into energy. Animal-based proteins are a source of niacin. Pellagra is a disease that results from a deficiency and consists of discolored, scaly skin, diarrhea, and mental confusion. I have also used this vitamin in certain types of hyperlipidemia with success, although it is limited in some patients due to the side effect of flushing.

Vitamin B6 supports the formation of blood cells and strengthens the immune system. It is also thought to ease the symptoms of morning sickness. Deficiency may include skin inflammation, depression, and irritability. Sources of vitamin B6 include poultry, beef, leafy green vegetables, and some fish. This vitamin has helped some patients who have cracks in the corners of their mouths.

Vitamin K plays a role in blood clotting and bone health. Sources include fruits, meat, and vegetables. Deficiencies can lead to increased bleeding. We need to carefully manipulate levels of this vitamin in patients with clotting issues.

Riboflavin, or vitamin B2, can be obtained from nuts, meat, milk, and green vegetables. It is required for proper development of blood cells, skin, and brain function. Patients sometimes use it to treat migraines and to lower homocysteine levels. High-dose ingestion can turn urine bright yellow.

Biotin, or vitamin B7, promotes the growth of hair and nails. This vitamin is found in eggs, nuts, and vegetables. In addition to brittle nails, a deficiency can cause rashes and neurological issues. I have often recommended this vitamin for nail and hair growth.

Vitamin B9 (synthetic form: leukovorin) is used to treat some forms of anemia, counteract toxic effects of other medications, and, according to a preliminary study, may be useful in patients with autism and cerebral folate deficiency.

Minerals play a role in structural support, enzymatic activity, nerve conduction and contraction, oxygen transport, immune function, DNA synthesis, and metabolic pathways. Chronic diseases, malabsorption, and drugs may all affect necessary nutrients and cause malnutrition. Patients with malnutrition are at high risk for multiple organ damage and mortality. Here is a rundown of essential minerals:

- Fluoride – Needed for bone and teeth structure. Deficiency leads to dental caries.
- Copper – Used in many enzyme reactions. Deficiency leads to anemia.
- Chromium – Helps potentiate insulin function. Deficiency leads to impaired glucose regulation.
- Pantothenic acid-
- Molybdenum – Co-factor for certain enzymes involved in sulfur metabolism.
- Selenium – Needed in many enzyme reactions. Deficiency can lead to cardiomyopathy.
- Zinc – Supports the immune system, aids in taste and smell, reproductive function, and DNA production. Deficiency leads to poor wound healing.
- Manganese – Helps form vitamin K. Deficiency can cause bleeding.
- Cobalt – Helps form blood cells. Deficiency can cause anemia.
- Silicon – Aids in bone production. Deficiency can lead to brittle nails and hair.
- Iron – Needed for hemoglobin production. Deficiency causes anemia.
- Iodine – Needed for thyroid hormone production. Deficiency results in hypothyroidism.

Not much is known about deficiencies of trace elements such as arsenic, nickel, tin, or vanadium.

Electrolytes (sodium, potassium, chloride, bicarbonate, calcium, magnesium) are minerals with an electrical charge and are responsible for bone health, neuromuscular function, and fluid and acid-base balance. Deficiencies can cause muscle cramping, twitching, irregular heartbeat, and metabolic issues.

CHAPTER 5

While nutrition plays a large part in healthy living, other areas of alternative treatment can play an important role as well. One of the most frequent modalities I have used in practice to give patients relief was ordering different types of physical therapy and exercise. Many times, therapy alleviated pain, improved quality of life, was cost-effective, and eliminated the use of drugs or surgery.

These modalities include stretching and strengthening exercises, balance and controlled gait training, massage, chiropractic manipulation, hydrotherapy, electrical stimulation, heat and ice therapy, speech therapy, and acupuncture. Studies indicate that adding chiropractic care to usual medical management results in a moderate short-term reduction in pain, reduced need for medications, and better patient satisfaction. Strengthening one's core through exercise is particularly helpful in chronic lower back pain.

As in many other medical conditions, education for prevention is important. Wearing proper sports equipment, using seatbelts, maintaining safe home and work spaces, engaging in regular exercise, using a cane if unsteady, and avoiding risky behavior can help keep you out of the hospital's emergency room.

I have also used acupuncture and dry needling with success in pain management conditions, especially neuropathic-type pain. The mechanism is not fully understood, but it can be a useful tool in nonpharmacological pain control. Acupuncture is a Chinese therapeutic technique that involves placing needles into specific areas of the body to stimulate nerves, muscles, and connective tissues. It is said to restore balance to the body's energy by unblocking channels through which Qi flows.

Similarly, TENS (transcutaneous electrical nerve stimulation) is a technique for pain relief that delivers electrical signals at pain sites. Studies suggest that the mechanism of action may involve modulation of neurotransmitter release and opioid activity.

Of note, studies show that mindfulness practices such as prayer, meditation, yoga, etc., are aids in nonpharmacological management of back pain. They are also extremely helpful in alleviating symptoms of anxiety and depression, again many times reducing the need for mood-modulating medications. They help individuals by promoting self-reflection, a sense of peace, emotional regulation, purpose, and relaxation. Prayer and meditation have been shown to lead to less depression and anxiety, improved coping with illness, and engagement in spiritual communities associated with lower mortality, less substance abuse, better mental health, and fewer depressive symptoms. Both practices may facilitate a restorative state that optimizes energy consumption and supports recovery from stress.

Many of these modalities result in the release of beneficial compounds termed exerkines, which have anti-inflammatory effects and help induce the release of antioxidant enzymes. They can modulate immune responses and affect hormonal and neurotransmitter pathways. These effects help reduce the risk of cardiac, metabolic, and neurological diseases.

Not only have I recommended these modalities for patients, but I am also able to speak from personal experience. As a result of an injury at a relatively young age, I was told multiple times that I had herniated disc disease and that I should consider surgical intervention. Instead, I perform a group of exercises known as

Williams flexion exercises, which are stretches and movements that strengthen core muscles. These exercises have saved me from having surgery, as they have done for many of my patients.

Studies have shown that exercising for 20 minutes per day provides significant health benefits, including reduced risk of all-cause mortality, improved cardiovascular and metabolic health, enhanced mental well-being, and increased life expectancy. This benefit applies across all age groups and sexes, even in patients with cardiovascular risk factors and metabolic issues.

CHAPTER 6

Herbs and supplements are used in many cultures for flavoring, perfume, and, for our purposes, health benefits. An herb, by definition, is a plant with seeds, leaves, or flowers that can be used for medicinal purposes. Dietary supplements are products that supplement the diet, such as vitamins, minerals, botanicals, amino acids, enzymes, and herbs.

We have reviewed some of these items previously, so we will now focus on herbal medicines. These remedies are not new; rather, some have been around for centuries. Evidence indicates that ancient civilizations self-medicated, and during the Greco-Roman era, Hippocrates started using herbs therapeutically in an orderly fashion. In the Golden Age, herbal medications were classified, and there has been a revival in modern times.

The list of herbs is extensive, and it is not my intent to list them all. If interested in a comprehensive catalog of herbs and supplements, I would suggest that the reader consult the PDR editions. In addition, herbalists sometimes form concoctions of various substances for specific diseases, which is beyond our scope here. Preparation may include oral forms such as capsules or tablets, infusions, ointments, poultices, oils, tinctures, etc.

We will go over some of the more common herbs and those that I have prescribed with some success. I will list them in groups to make them easier to remember. I will also attempt to give a description of each herb, which I have gathered from various internet sources, since I am not a botanist and, like most consumers, am reliant on commercial products.

Some of the most frequent complaints of patients who came to the office were anxiety and depression. Herbs that are helpful for these conditions include kava, lavender, passion flower, lemon balm, ashwagandha, St. John's wort, curcumin, valerian, chamomile, saffron, black cohosh, chasteberry, and skullcap. Chamomile tea was especially helpful for patients having difficulty sleeping.

ANXIETY / DEPRESSION

Chamomile is a daisy-like flowering plant known for its soothing effect and apple-like scent. It has anti-inflammatory and antioxidant effects. It also exhibits anxiolytic and sedative properties and is helpful in easing digestive complaints. There is also some antibacterial activity. Chamomile is relatively safe, but allergic reactions can occur, and it may interact with certain medications such as anticoagulants and CNS or psychotropic medications. It is available as a tea, capsule, or topical preparation (for eczema).

Kava is made from the root of a plant in the pepper family. It has demonstrated short-term reduction in anxiety and restlessness. Adverse reactions include headache, cognitive impairment, and tremor. Liver dysfunction has been reported, so liver function should be monitored with more chronic use. It is available as a tea or extract.

Lavender is a fragrant flowering plant known for its soothing scent. Oral preparations, as well as inhalation of lavender essential oil, have been shown to reduce anxiety. It is helpful in improving sleep quality and may possess some pain-relieving properties. Occasional skin dermatitis may occur, but overall, the safety profile is good. It is available in capsules and tinctures.

Passion flower is a fast-growing climbing vine known for its star-shaped flowers and edible fruit. Most evidence supports its use in anxiety reduction and sleep improvement. This plant is generally well tolerated and is available as a capsule or tincture.

Lemon balm is a bushy plant with heart-shaped leaves and small white or pink flowers. It is used in aromatherapy for its calming effect. It has antianxiety and antidepressant qualities. It may also enhance sleep and improve cognitive function. It is generally well tolerated and available as a tea, lip ointment, or tincture.

Ashwagandha is an evergreen shrub also known as winter cherry or Indian ginseng. It is useful in stress reduction, sleep improvement, and cognitive function. It also exhibits anti-inflammatory, antioxidant, and immunomodulatory properties. There is some evidence that it helps normalize certain hormones. It is usually safe, although occasional gastrointestinal symptoms, somnolence, or allergic reactions may occur. It is available as a tea, capsule, or tincture.

St. John's wort is an herb known for its bright yellow, five-petaled flowers with translucent dots. Its primary health benefit is in the treatment of depression. It is generally well-tolerated but can cause gastrointestinal distress. One of its major limitations is that it is a potent inducer of cytochrome enzymes, which can cause interactions with many medications. It is available as a tea, capsule, or tincture.

Curcumin comes from the underground stem of an East Indian plant. This herb has health benefits in chronic inflammatory conditions. I have listed it here because of its use as an herb that may help with depression. It is usually well tolerated in normal doses and is available as a tea, capsule, or extract.

Valerian is a fragrant plant with white to pink flowers and a pungent-smelling root. It is helpful in improving sleep in patients with insomnia and in decreasing anxiety. It is usually well tolerated but can cause headache or mild gastrointestinal distress. It is available as tea, extract, or capsules.

Saffron is a spice derived from the flower of Crocus sativus. Its potential benefit is improving mood and alleviating anxiety and depression, possibly by affecting brain chemicals such as serotonin and dopamine. It may also reduce symptoms of premenstrual syndrome and improve sexual function in men. It is available in capsule form, powders, liquid extracts, and gummies.

Black cohosh is a plant known for its tall spires of white flowers and green foliage. It is thought to help alleviate menopausal symptoms such as hot flashes and mood swings. Black cohosh does not have an estrogenic effect on the breast or endometrium and is usually well tolerated. It is available as a tea, capsule, or tincture.

Chasteberry, derived from the fruit of the chaste tree, is helpful for menstrual irregularities, premenstrual syndrome, and breast pain. It is usually well tolerated, with minor adverse effects such as dry mouth, gastrointestinal complaints, or dizziness. It is available as a tea, capsule, or extract.

Skullcap is a plant in the mint family with helmet-shaped flowers and square stems. It has some anti-inflammatory and antioxidant properties and is thought to be helpful for cognitive enhancement, anxiety, and depression. It is generally well tolerated, but quality control is important, as serious adverse reactions have occurred with adulterated products. It is available as a tea, capsule, or tablet.

Other than prescription medications, I have used chamomile (for sleep), black cohosh (for menopausal symptoms), and lavender and kava (for anxiety) with some success. I have avoided St. John's wort due to its potential drug interactions.

CHAPTER 7

Another common complaint in the office involves respiratory infections. Some are bacterial, but the majority are viral. The advent of in-office testing has been helpful in detecting streptococcal infections, COVID infections, and influenza, to mention a few. Inappropriate antibiotic use for viruses is not only unnecessary but may be harmful. Many times, symptomatic treatment is helpful and all that is required. In this area, certain herbs may be helpful along with home remedies. This group includes peppermint, eucalyptus, licorice root, ginger, thyme, oregano, elderberry, andrographis, pelargonium, ivy leaf extract, mullein, and echinacea.

RESPIRATORY SYMPTOMS

Peppermint is an herb known for its strong minty flavor and aroma due to its high menthol content. It has smooth, dark green leaves and stems with a purple tinge. It is helpful in digestive complaints such as bloating, upset stomach, and nausea, and is used in aromatherapy as an oil to help breathing and break up mucus.

Eucalyptus is a fast-growing tree with distinctive bark and aromatic leaves due to the oil glands it contains. The flowers may form a cap. This herb is used in essential oils, creams, and lozenges to help with cough, congestion, and muscle aches, as it has some anti-inflammatory properties. Gargling with the leaves may soothe sore throats. It is also used in tea form to help with bronchitis or may be given as a capsule or applied to the chest in ointment form.

Licorice is used for mouth ulcers, laryngitis, and cough. It comes in lozenges, tea, and tablet forms. This plant can grow tall with leaflets that produce blue, sweet pea–like flowers. The roots are processed to make licorice and black sugar. Long-term use can affect potassium levels.

Ginger is a flowering plant with a knobby-shaped root and various colored flowers. In addition to its culinary uses, it has health benefits that include alleviation of nausea and constipation. It is a natural antiviral and anti-inflammatory, which may reduce inflammation in the respiratory tract and act as a cough suppressant. It is available in capsule and tea form and as an essential oil, which is used for some skin irritations and to promote hair growth. Care must be taken in patients on anticoagulation.

Thyme is a low-growing shrub with oval leaves that contain an oil thought to have antiseptic properties. Herbalists use thyme for colds and influenza. Its antispasmodic effect makes it useful in asthma and bronchitis. It is available as a tea, capsule, or syrup. The side effect profile is generally benign.

Oregano is a perennial herb that grows as a bushy plant with small oval green leaves and white or pink flowers. It has antibacterial, antifungal, antiviral, and anti-inflammatory properties, making it helpful in fighting infections. It is available as a tea or oil. Patients taking lithium should avoid oregano.

Elderberry is a fast-growing shrub with clusters of white flowers, serrated leaves, and dark purple berries. It is used to treat colds and influenza and is available as a syrup or lozenge. The berries can be eaten but must be cooked first. Care should be taken in patients with an altered immune status.

Andrographis is an annual herb with a dark green quadrangular stem, smooth leaves, and white flowers with purple spots on the petals. It is used to reduce fever and treat colds, influenza, and bronchitis. It is available as capsules, tablets, or liquid extracts. Side effects are usually mild, with gastrointestinal symptoms being the most common.

Pelargonium, also known as geranium, is a flowering plant whose blossoms resemble a stork's beak and have scented leaves. Herbalists use it as a lozenge, extract, or tincture to reduce symptoms of cough, colds, sore throat, and bronchitis. It is usually well tolerated, though occasional rash or stomach upset may occur.

Ivy leaf is a green climbing plant that contains saponins, flavonoids, and phenolic acids. It acts as an expectorant and has anti-inflammatory effects. It is available as a syrup or tincture. Adverse reactions are rare but may include occasional gastrointestinal symptoms.

Mullein is a plant known for its tall, fuzzy stalks and yellow flowers. It is rich in mucilage, which can soothe the throat, and saponins, which help loosen congestion. The seeds are toxic and should not be ingested. When used in tea form, the fine hairs can be irritating, so they should be strained out before drinking. It is useful in respiratory infections due to its anti-inflammatory and expectorant qualities and is usually well-tolerated.

Echinacea is a wildflower with a daisy-like bloom and a prominent central cone that can be purple, white, red, orange, or yellow. It is rich in antioxidants and used as a remedy for colds and influenza. It is available in tablets, tinctures, extracts, and tea. The plant contains caffeic acid, alkamides, phenolic acids, rosmarinic acid, and polyacetylenes, which help enhance immunity and reduce inflammation. It is usually well tolerated, though occasional rash or gastrointestinal symptoms may occur.

My most frequently used herbs in this area were echinacea and eucalyptus.

CHAPTER 8

CNS MODULATION

Several herbs have demonstrated central nervous system health benefits, especially in neuroprotection and cognitive enhancement. We have already mentioned some herbs that help with anxiety and depression, such as sage, rosemary, and lavender. Others, such as ginkgo biloba, bacopa monnieri, and Panax ginseng, have additional neuroprotective effects and may improve cognitive functioning. In addition, green tea has shown some evidence for memory improvement.

Ginkgo biloba is an ancient tree with unique fan-shaped leaves and produces a foul-smelling fruit (non-edible). Its leaves are used to boost cognitive function due to their antioxidant properties. It can be used in capsule, extract, tea, or tincture form. Side effects include increased risk of bleeding, interaction with certain antidepressant medications, allergic reactions, and possible gastrointestinal symptoms. In this class, this was the most common herb that I recommended, with limited improvement seen.

Bacopa monnieri is a plant that contains compounds such as alkaloids, saponins, and cucurbitacins thought to have memory-enhancing properties. The leaves are oblong and thick, and the flowers are small and white to purple with four or five petals. It is available as tea, infusion, extract, or capsule. It is usually well tolerated, though occasional gastrointestinal side effects may occur. There can be drug interactions with this herb.

Panax ginseng has a thick, fleshy root that is brown or yellow. The active ingredients are ginsenosides, which have antioxidant, anti-inflammatory, and immune-enhancing effects. It is thought that taking Panax ginseng by mouth may improve cognitive function. It is available as a capsule or extract. It is relatively safe when taken short-term, though uncommon side effects include severe rash and liver damage. This herb interacts with Coumadin and some other medications.

Many herbs have been used for various medical conditions due to their anti-inflammatory and antioxidant properties. In addition to chamomile, garlic, and ginger previously mentioned, some of the better-known ones are curcumin, soursop, nigella sativa, willow bark, and pomegranate.

CHAPTER 9

ANTI-INFLAMMATORY HERBS

One of the best-known herbs in this group is turmeric, whose nutritional compound is curcumin, a bright yellow substance with anti-inflammatory and antioxidant properties. Due to its ability to reduce inflammation and oxidation, this substance is felt to lower the risk of heart disease. It is also thought to be helpful in conditions where chronic inflammation exists, such as arthritis, certain gastrointestinal conditions, skin conditions, lung conditions, and mental health conditions. Generally well tolerated, but it can interfere with some medications. Available in capsule, liquid, and powder forms.

Soursop is a tropical fruit tree whose fruit, leaves, bark, and seeds have demonstrated anticancer activity due to its compound annonaceous acetogenins, antioxidant and anti-inflammatory activity due to quercetin and kaempferol, and also antimicrobial, analgesic, and metabolic effects. It is usually well tolerated, except that neurotoxicity has been reported in animal models. Available as juice, capsules, tea extract, and drops.

Nigella sativa is a flowering plant with anti-inflammatory and antioxidant effects. It contains thymoquinone, flavonoids, and unsaturated fatty acids and is helpful in a number of respiratory, inflammatory, and endocrine conditions. Available in powder, capsule, and liquid forms. Usually safe but may interact with blood thinners.

Willow bark is the bark from several willow trees and contains a compound called salicin, which the body converts to salicylic acid, the same chemical that was used to develop aspirin. It also contains flavonoids and polyphenols contributing to its anti-inflammatory and antioxidant properties. It is used in inflammatory conditions and in skin care products. Care should be taken in cases of aspirin allergy and with bleeding risk. Available as tea, powder, liquid, and capsule forms.

Pomegranate is rich in ellagitannins, anthocyanins, and polyphenols, which can help protect against cell damage and have a beneficial effect in conditions such as arthritis and heart disease. It is a large shrub with glossy, lance-shaped leaves and large red or white flowers that develop into fruit. Available as a fruit or in liquid form. Usually well tolerated, with only occasional gastrointestinal symptoms being reported.

The most common herb that I had recommended in this group was turmeric to decrease inflammation and thereby give some relief of discomfort if medication was not warranted, and pomegranates for heart health.

CHAPTER 10

The next group relates to women's and men's health.

MEN

Saw palmetto is a small, slow-growing palm tree. It has a saw-toothed stem and fan-shaped leaves. It produces small berry-like fruits that are used medicinally to help reduce symptoms of benign prostatic hypertrophy. The active ingredients are liposterols. It is available as a capsule or tablet, and side effects are usually minimal.

Nettle is a plant with serrated leaves and needle-sharp hairs. Used in contact with painful areas, it can act almost like dry needling and provide some pain relief. Uses also include hay fever and arthritis, but it is used to alleviate the symptoms of benign prostatic hypertrophy. Available as a capsule, tea, and extract. It can interfere with certain medications and occasionally cause rash, gastrointestinal upset, and sexual dysfunction.

WOMEN

Soy is a plant-based food that is the product of the soybean plant. It contains all of the essential amino acids, has a number of vitamins and minerals, and contains isoflavones and phytoestrogens, which are antioxidants and have estrogen-like activity. It is the latter that gives it usefulness in alleviating menopausal symptoms such as sweating and hot flashes. The plant has oval leaflets and small white flowers. The fruit is in a covered pod. Available as a food. There may be some interactions with certain medications.

The other herb that I had found useful in helping to alleviate menopausal symptoms is black cohosh, which has been described previously.

CHAPTER 11

MISCELLANEOUS HERBAL EFFECTS

Hops, known for their use in brewing beer, are helpful in digestion and sedation. Available as a supplement or tea.

Butterbur, useful in seasonal allergies and for migraine prevention. It causes less drowsiness than many classical cold medications. Available as capsules, tablets, powder, and tinctures.

Goldenseal, known for its distinctive thick, bright yellow stem, which has compounds that are used to treat the common cold and also help digestion. Available as a capsule, tea, and, due to antimicrobial effects, as a topical and mouthwash (for mouth ulcers). Not recommended in pregnancy and may interfere with some medications.

Cinnamon, contains polyphenols that help control blood sugar. Available as a capsule, tea, and powder. Ceylon cinnamon is promoted for allergic rhinitis and is also used in topical form as a mosquito repellent.

Psyllium, because of its rich fiber content, psyllium is used to relieve constipation and may be helpful in lowering cholesterol, helping with heart health. Available as a powder and capsule.

Peppermint, a combination of watermint and spearmint, this herb is used in culinary, medicinal, and cosmetic applications. Taken orally, it helps with digestion in conditions such as irritable bowel and can be used locally to reduce pain and itching. Available as a tea, capsule, and ointment.

Feverfew, available as a capsule, this herb is known to treat migraine headaches.

Hibiscus, in addition to containing antioxidants, this herb has diuretic properties and is helpful in lowering blood pressure. Available in capsule and tea forms.

Milk Thistle, known to detoxify the liver due to compounds known as flavonolignans. Available in capsule, extract, tablet, and tea forms.

Cat's Claw, named for its hooked thorns, contains antioxidants and anti-inflammatory compounds, which make it helpful in treating various types of arthritis. Available as a capsule, extract, and tea.

CHAPTER 12

We have discussed the benefits of diet, exercise, vitamins, minerals, and herbs on healthy aging, but there are other factors to consider in longevity and healthy aging, one of the most important of which is genetics. This is an area where both alternative therapy and modern medicine may play a role.

Our body is made up of trillions of cells. The genetic material inside those cells determines which function a particular cell will become. Many cells start as undifferentiated (stem) cells, and specific foci on our genes are responsible for differentiating these cells into different organ cells, while others are responsible for repair and regeneration. Telomeres are at the end of chromosomes and shorten with cell division, thought to encourage cell aging. Environmental factors can damage DNA or disrupt regulatory pathways and lead to aging. Certain changes in the DNA and cell structures can occur with aging and thereby limit the ability to produce stem cells for regeneration or cause them to be dysfunctional. This has led to some patients paying for stem cell therapy for various conditions and attempting to retard the aging process. The process is costly and not practical for most people. Conversely, a healthy lifestyle, positive thoughts, and stress management with practices such as meditation can help produce an enzyme that helps in cell regeneration and protection.

There are also some herbs that influence stem cell production and function. Polyphenols and phytochemicals from plants, including ginseng, resveratrol, curcumin, epigallocatechin gallate, genistein, naringin, icariin, astragalus, angelica, as well as blueberries, green tea, and a number of traditional Chinese herbs such as Radix Astragali, Herba Epimedii, Saussurea involucrata, Withania somnifera, and Tinospora cordifolia, have been shown to increase proliferation and delay senescence. Of note, there is no FDA-approved herb for this indication as of yet.

On the medical side, CRISPR therapy is a gene-editing approach that uses systems to make precise, permanent changes to DNA in living cells and is presently being used as treatment in some human genetic diseases. Although it is presently not recognized as an anti-aging therapy, it has shown promise in age-related conditions. It is my opinion that with the refinement of gene sequencing and their products that regulate the cell by quantum and supercomputers, there will be tremendous breakthroughs that will represent the future of modern medicine.

CHAPTER 13

We start to see a shift from mystical treatments to observation, clinical experience, prognosis, and the healing power of nature in Ancient Greece, especially with the work of Hippocrates. This philosophy developed throughout the ages into many traditional therapies, some of which we have discussed. Although complex, large-scale improvements were not seen or documented using traditional medicine alone.

It was not until the late 19th to early 20th century, with the advent of anesthetics, X-rays, scientific theory, germ theory, sanitation, public health measures, antibiotics, vaccines, and better treatment for chronic conditions such as diabetes, heart, lung, and kidney disease with pharmaceuticals and devices, that a significant improvement in mortality occurred.

Let's start with the introduction of antibiotics in the 1930s and 1940s. With their discovery and usage, there was a dramatic reduction in human mortality. Before antibiotics, diseases such as pneumonia, sepsis, and tuberculosis were some of the leading causes of death worldwide. With the widespread clinical usage of penicillin and sulfonamides, along with improvements in nutrition, public health initiatives, and sanitation, lifespan was significantly improved on average. Unfortunately, drug resistance is becoming more prevalent, requiring stewardship and innovation for newer antibiotics, which are more expensive and may have additional side effects. With the advent of vaccines, many diseases were eliminated or contained.

Next, let's look at the improvement of cardiac care and stroke over the past century. The combination of newer medications, surgical procedures, stenting, coronary care units, thrombolysis, and risk factor management (smoking cessation, hypertension, and cholesterol control) has increased life expectancy dramatically. Although, as of this date, no stem cell therapy has become standard of care in ischemic heart disease and heart failure, it is investigational and represents an exciting possibility for future care.

Cancer care has reduced human mortality significantly over the past century due to advances in treatment, earlier detection, and prevention. Surgery, radiotherapy, chemotherapy, targeted therapies, and immunotherapies have been major contributors to this decline. In addition, prevention such as smoking cessation and limiting alcohol consumption, as well as early detection by screening, have played a role. Again, stem cells play multiple roles in cancer treatment. They are used in cancer therapy for tissue regeneration, as innovative drug delivery systems, and as key targets for novel therapies.

Another factor causing deaths in humans is related to mental illness and substance abuse. While some advances have been made, the overall impact on population-level mortality rates has been limited, and these groups continue to experience elevated mortality rates and reduced life expectancy compared to the general public. This is an area where both traditional and modern medicine can help with supplements, medication, and interventions, but it is only the individual who can decide to make a difference.

Likewise, individuals can impact another significant contributor to their own mortality, namely unintentional injuries caused by accidents. For many years, I had lectured our elderly patients about getting up on step stools or chairs due to their fall risk. Many who did not heed that advice ended up in the hospital with fractures, which at times led to their death. Also, keeping their environment clutter-free significantly lessens the chances of falling. When gait instability was present for any reason, we would aggressively argue for gait training and core strengthening for fall prevention.

We would try to counsel our younger patients against speeding or driving under the influence to prevent car accidents and to wear proper equipment when engaging in sports activities. We would explain the complications of drug addiction or unintentional poisonings to our patient population in an effort to reduce drug overdoses, a major cause of mortality. Safety around water activities can prevent drownings. Proper firearm storage and safety were stressed.

These groups of unintentional injuries represent a major contributor to global mortality, with estimates of 1.8 million deaths annually and billions in health care costs.

Finally, studies have demonstrated that loneliness is a significant factor for all-cause mortality. This effect occurs slightly more in men and most likely happens through pathways of mental health, functional decline, and biological aging. Cognitive behavioral therapy and community engagement programs can be effective, and I have witnessed the value of owning and caring for a pet in this regard.

So back to my original question: Can one's aging and time of death be affected by an individual's actions, or is it a clock with no snooze button? I have attempted to show some of the variables that humans do have under their control, starting with what's on their plate, exercise, meditation and prayer, safety issues, regular checkups, avoiding destructive behaviors, sleep hygiene, supplements, vitamins, avoiding unnecessary medications and vaccines but taking proper pharmaceuticals and vaccinations, and being socially engaged. These can affect not only the quality of how we live in our later years but also extend that "time."

www.ingramcontent.com/pod-product-compliance
Lightning Source LLC
Chambersburg PA
CBHW051337150726
47997CB00004B/1502